Anti Inflammatory Diet

I0410525

Know Everything About Inflammation & Ways To Control It

Written by

Cheryl Barnhart

Cheryl Barnhart

photocopy, recording, or any information storage or retrieval system, without permission in writing from the publisher.

No responsibility or liability is assumed by the Publisher for any injury, damage or financial loss sustained to persons or property from the use of this information, personal or otherwise, either directly or indirectly. While every effort has been made to ensure reliability and accuracy of the information within, all liability, negligence or otherwise, from any use, misuse or abuse of the operation of any methods, strategies, instructions or ideas contained in the material herein, is the sole responsibility of the reader.

Any copyrights not held by publisher are owned by their respective authors.

All information is generalized, presented for informational purposes only and presented

ACKNOWLEDGMENTS

For my students and friends, who all selflessly helped me in writing this book. Special thanks to those who asked, insisted and assisted me in turning the seminars in this practical form. All Rights Reserved 2012-2015 @ Cheryl Barnhart

TABLE OF CONTENT

INTRODUCTION

From the very first day after birth and along the whole life, our body gets vulnerable to chemicals, toxins, bacteria, viruses, and various threatening factors. Luckily, our body initiates inflammation to combat these adverse situations. These threats are removed properly and promptly with this inflammatory response.

According to years of research, inflammatory response is not always good to our body. It also leads to several inflammatory diseases. Most of us venture through "silent" inflammation which can adversely affect our body. Inflammation suddenly becomes the evil instead of healing and protecting the body. The causes of inflammation can easily be seen with the increased risk of diabetes, heart disease, Alzheimer's disease, cancer, and autoimmune diseases.

What if Good Things in Our Body Turn Evil?

Especially in medical science, the most common option is to address the disease, symptoms, and conditions with prescription drugs and over-the-counter medications. But it will treat inflammation on temporary basis. In this book, we are going to discuss inflammation and its causes and the natural and safe ways to permanently cure inflammation.

Here, we will discuss how lifestyle and diet chances can affect inflammation and prevent several inflammatory diseases consequently. A lot of studies have suggested the diets that can trigger the inflammation of body. This "Anti-Inflammatory Diet" guide will help you know how inflammation works so you can better control your internal inflammatory environment. This guide will help you target vulnerability and inflammatory touch points and make a plan to keep the inflammation at bay. You will also learn preparing some healthy and delicious foods to treat inflammation and live a fulfilling and happy life.

CHAPTER 1

WHAT IS INFLAMMATION?

Suppose you found the way to make some lifestyle changes and avoid lots of health issues like stroke, heart disease, Alzheimer's disease, diabetes, and arthritis. Would you like to go for it? This chapter will explain what inflammation is, the connection between inflammation and diseases and the ways to reduce and prevent inflammation with various lifestyle and diet changes.

Inflammation is considered as the leading cause of several diseases that can make us depressed and cut our lifespan. But the best thing is that you can control and avoid several health issues by controlling your inflammation and starting an anti-inflammatory diet. With this diet, you won't be able to prevent any specific disease. In fact, you will be controlling all the unhealthy factors.

Here, you will be able to learn what inflammation is, how it is responsible for causing several diseases and the relation between CRP and inflammation.

What Is Inflammation?

Usually, inflammation is a healing, defensive element. It protects our body from several viral elements. For example, if you suddenly cut your hand, if any part of the body is burned, or if virus enters your body, these molecules prevent infection from our body. They "lock" the wound area down for healing and to avoid infection.

*Simply put, **inflammation** is a body's defense against chemical reactions, infection, and allergies. Some of the* *common reactions are heat, swelling, pain and redness and any part may be inflamed.*

Once the threat is gone and the attack is over, inflammation naturally gets back to its normal state and is prepared to avoid another attack. Sometimes, inflammation doesn't depart and this schedule crashes. It leads to prolonged problem that worsen eventually. Excess body fat, saturated fats, too much smoking and several assaults cause inflammation for a long time that is quiet, but chronic.

This silent, low-grade inflammation can intruder without any cause. It occurs without even giving any sign and causes several health conditions.

Symptoms of Inflammation

Inflammation causes several serious problems and it is a common thread and some of these problems are chronic. Here are some of the serious health conditions caused by inflammation –

- Diabetes
- Cancer, heart stroke and heart disease – the major killers in the US
- Inflammatory bowel disease (Crohn's Disease and Ulcerative Colitis)
- Lupus and Rheumatoid Arthritis – Some of the common types of arthritis
- Acne
- Allergies
- Other autoimmune issues like multiple sclerosis and lupus.

According to the affect area of your body, symptoms of inflammation may vary. For example, inflammation may develop atherosclerosis in your blood vessels. If it is your case, you might face a heart attack. Or you might twist or fall your ankle that may swell, turn red or hurt.

Why Is Inflammation Responsible For All Serious Age-Related Problems?

According to recent researches, wrinkling skin, losing away muscle, and high chances of chronic and acute disease and several inevitable reasons of aging are caused by inflammation. In fact, you can reduce the signs of aging by reducing inflammation. According to Claudio Franceschi, an Italian researcher, aging is strongly connected inflammation and this process is called as "inflammaging". It is the most important and common reason of age-related problems.

According to Dr. Caleb Finch from the University of Southern California, people had longer lifespan in the last century than today because they were less prone to infectious diseases and various inflammation sources. So, it is recommended to have anti-inflammatory diet to reverse back the signs of aging.

Inflammation & CRP

How would you determine how much your body is inflamed? There is an affordable blood test with which both your doctor and you can find out the levels of inflammation in your body.

CRP or **C - reactive protein** is found in the blood whose level drastically increases when inflammation grows in your body. It is also known to work as an advance defense system against infections. CRP tests are not new and doctors have done it for several years to determine the level of inflammation in patients who have rheumatoid arthritis, lupus, and various inflammatory diseases. In several studies, the relation between heart disease and CRP levels has been shown.

The Source of CRP

CRP is normally grown by the fat around the area of stomach and liver. It is produced between two arteries through which blood is supplied to your heart.

According to blood tests, if cholesterol level is found normal or below 200 mg/dl, don't believe that you cannot have heart disease in future. Despite of cholesterol levels, if you are found with high CRP levels, you are also prone to heart problems like strokes and heart attacks. According to lifestyle and genetic history, the level of CRP produced by the body varies according to the person. If you don't exercise, are overweight, smoke or have high BP, the CRP levels might be high. On the flip side, the CRP levels might be low if you are athletic and lean.

CHAPTER 2

WHAT IF INFLAMMATION GOES OUT OF CONTROL?

From head to toe, inflammation is related partly, or completely, with different types of diseases. It may also go out of control and cause critical illnesses. Inflammation is covered in several diseases which may lead to serious disability like stroke, heart disease, diabetes, cancer and Alzheimer's disease. Here, you will be able to learn about some diseases that can be caused by inflammation – some are milder which can cause serious health problems while some are dangerous.

Inflammation Causes Heart Attacks

Usually heart attack is responsible for large number of deaths in the world.

Heart disease is normally caused when the blood vessels are clogged through which the blood is supplied to your heart.

> **Did You Know?**
> Our arteries transfer oxygen-rich blood to our body tissues. The deposits of fatty material, plaques, can easily build up within the walls of artery. Atherosclerotic Plaques cause inflammatory reactions on the innermost layer of artery walls. These plaques narrow down the arteries and cause blood clots. As a result, it leads to heart problems.

Atherosclerosis stores large number of CRP levels and it is known to cause heart disease. Higher CRP levels mean higher risk of having stroke or heart disease. CRP refers are widely referred to as an inflammatory "marker" by the physicians. High-sensitivity CRP test has been recommended by most doctors today if patient develops heart disease, stroke or any health condition related to inflammation. In this test, how much your body is inflamed can be measured.

In order to determine the process related to Atherosclerosis, a clogged plumbing analogy is used by the scientists and media. According to them, the bad cholesterol levels (also known as "LDL Cholesterol") clog the pipes and turn down the blood circulation.

According to the scientists, blood vessels are thin tubes of living, narrow tissue. LDL Cholesterol damages the walls of the artery and causes the injury that leads to inflammation. As a result, the protective cells start their work. But they change and enlarge LDL cholesterol deposits and turn them into plaques. Other molecules weaken up the cap on the top of plaque. The cap eventually bursts and the plaque contents make another mess and leads to a huge blood clot, stroke or heart attack.

Symptoms of Heart Disease

Squeezing, Chest Pain (Angina), pain at the center of chest, fullness and pain on neck, shoulders or arms are some of the common signs. Women may also have some unusual signs like dizziness, upset stomach; shortness of breath, rapid heartburns and fatigue. Sometimes, you may have none of such symptoms, while some people have most of them.

Inflammation Causes Alzheimer's Disease

Inflammation also has connection with chronic brain diseases like Alzheimer's disease. According to the researches, the brain cells can be destroyed by chronic inflammation and it attacks nerve cells and both of them cause dementia. Neurologists are still working to determine the actual cause of Alzheimer's disease. According to them, the immune cells of the body attack the brain's beta-amyloidal proteins. These proteins usually live in your brain and are not harmful at all. When these proteins become plaques because of inflammation, they cause cognitive problems. These plaques are known to build up in your brain and cause Alzheimer's disease.

There is a brain constituent named "Tao Protein" that maintains nerve structure. According to the researchers, people who have Alzheimer's disease may normally have twisted Tao protein which can cause nerve damage. The brain stops functioning well when damaged neurons start increasing in the brain.

It is believed that these plaques and inflammation are commonly related with Alzheimer's disease and may cause common infections to the individual. The plaques affect those parts of your brain which help in thinking, decision-making and memory.

Luckily you can take control on dementia and Alzheimer's disease with anti-inflammatory food. Start having brain-healthy diet which has limited

Trans Fats and saturated fats. Increase eating vegetables and fruits. According to researches, the photochemical can keep free radicals from damaging brain cells and reduce the growth of such plaques. This way, you need to eat those vegetables and fruits that make up rainbow colors like yellow, red, orange etc. For example, eggplant, oranges, beets, orange bell peppers, cherries, eggplants and various berries.

Certain omega-3 rich foods can also work as dietary support to prevent Alzheimer's. They maintain brain cells well and reduce the risk of Alzheimer's disease by 60%.

Other Diseases Caused by Inflammation

Although Alzheimer's disease and heart attack are the major causes of inflammation, there are some other diseases you should beware of because they are also caused by inflammation.

Cancer

Cancer is another great fear which occurs in different areas of your body with several symptoms. Cancer is of different types, say cervical, breast, liver, ovarian, pancreatic and urinary bladder and all of them are connected to inflammation. According to recent researches, most of the cancerous and precancerous cells have common signs of inflammation. It is also proved that inflammation can lead to higher risk of developing cancer.

Stroke

When the bleeding or blood clot suddenly stops the blood circulation in brain, the inflammation causes stroke. It is often called as brain attacks. When brain cells stop functioning and get deprived of blood, strokes are known to occur. The brain cells die if bleeding continues for longer time.

Here are some of the alarming symptoms of stroke –

- Trouble understanding, speaking or sudden confusion
- Sudden weakness or numbness of arm, face, leg, or one side of your body
- Severe, sudden headache without any cause
- Dizziness, trouble walking, loss of coordination or balance all of a sudden
- Sudden loss of vision from one or both eyes

Diabetes

Inflammation in blood vessels causes diabetes and it also leads to cause stroke and heart disease. According to a study, women who were found with inflamed blood vessels were 5 times more prone to Type II diabetes than others.

Did You Know?
Over 17 Million people in the US have diabetes
In the US alone, the cases of diabetes rose up by 50% over the past decade
One in three people born in the US in 2000 might develop diabetes.

The person suffering from diabetes may develop a threatening level of sugar in the blood. When body becomes unable to produce insulin to transform food into energy, you may develop Type II diabetes which can be life-threatening and serious. Diabetes may lead to nerve damage, blindness, heart disease, and kidney issues. So, it is good to start a healthy anti-inflammatory diet to control everything that can be caused by diabetes.

CHAPTER 3

ANTI-INFLAMMATORY DIET

Anti-inflammatory diet is as valuable as diet for weight loss or heart health. If you have successfully maintained your immune system, it will help reduce inflammation. It will not just prevent autoimmune disorders, but it will also help you combat diabetes, heart disease and Alzheimer's disease. It is similar to any other healthy diet. But it includes some specific nutrients which are helpful to control inflammation.

How it is Beneficial?

Since inflammation is prone to increase or decrease due to certain diet or food intake, it is very important to choose anti-inflammatory foods that can help control risk of several health issues, such as heart disease, Alzheimer's disease, psoriasis, diabetes, Crohn's disease, and rheumatoid arthritis.

Antioxidants Control Inflammation

There are certain vegetables and fruits that provide antioxidants of high amounts to control inflammation. There are some plant chemicals like flavonoids and beta-carotene which are really very beneficial. These foods also contain Vitamin A, C and E. Choose fruits and vegetables of bright color because they have more antioxidants than less-colorful ones. Have several colored veggies and fruits every week, such as berries, cherries, grapes, green leafy vegetables, sweet potatoes and carrots. All of them are nutritious. Eat about 3 servings of fruits and 4 servings of veggies every day.

Fiber-Rich Whole Grains Help in Arthritis

There are some foods which have refined grains. Whole grains have antioxidants which are rich in fiber. Some of the rich sources are oatmeal, whole-wheat bread, whole-wheat pasta and brown rice that can help you in anti-inflammatory diet. According to the Arthritis Foundation, it is important to eat at least 2 to 3 servings of pasta every week and whole grains of at least 3 to 5 servings every day to reduce inflammation.

Protein Foods

This way, you need to choose plant-based sources of protein like seeds, nuts, and beans and some of the animal-based sources of protein, such as salmon, sardines and other omega-3 rich fish. Other rich sources of protein are cheese, eggs, lean meat, yogurt and poultry. But you should eat these foods less often, i.e.

for around once or twice a week as they have saturated fats that can improve inflammation.

Healthy Fats Also Reduce Inflammation

Fats are also healthy if they are taken from Omega-3 acids and monounsaturated fats. They both can help reduce inflammation. Avoid taking fat from Omega-6 and saturated fats. Some of the rich sources of Omega-3 fats are walnuts, fatty fish and flaxseeds and some of the rich sources of monounsaturated fats are seeds, nuts, olive oil and avocados. These foods will help you improve good cholesterol levels and reduce inflammation.

Other Healthy Sources

There are some herbs and spices and tea which are rich in antioxidants and they have great anti-inflammatory effect.

Make sure not to add sugar and cream on your tea. There are some simple carbohydrates found in sugar can increase blood sugar levels which may promote inflammation. You can add the flavorings in your foods with oregano, rosemary, curry, ginger, dill and cinnamon in place of salt. If you want to reduce severe inflammation, you can add chili peppers, garlic and turmeric on your food.

Why to Adopt It?

The Anti-Inflammatory Diet is based on foods which are healthy sources of Omega-3 acids, polyphenols, Vitamins C and E, probiotics and prebiotics which can reduce inflammation. In order to get essential vital nutrients, you need to eat vegetables and fruits, legumes, whole grains and fatty fish like tuna and salmon and healthy fats like avocados and olive oil. Add cherries and berries in your diet to intake pole phenols. Add a lot of nutrient-dense vegetables like leafy greens. Use spices and herbs to add flavors.

In order to reduce inflammation, control the intake of unhealthy and saturated foods. Also avoid foods rich in Trans Fats and refined carbs like baked foods and fast foods which have saturated fat like bacon and butter.

Anti Inflammatory Diet Principles

Breakfast

Start up your day with immunity-boosting, healthy breakfast, like oatmeal, walnuts, blueberries and chia seeds. Add these ingredients to your bowl and have a cup of almond or soy milk or nonfat milk. You can also make a healthy and tasty anti-inflammatory breakfast with an omelet with toasted English whole-wheat muffin and spinach or a bowl of cantaloupe and mashed avocado.

You can also blend bananas, strawberries, Greek yogurt and flax oil for on-the-go nutrient-rich breakfast flaxseeds, Chia seeds and walnuts have omega-3 acids.

Lunch

Have vegetables and fruits which can help you get all the essential nutrients for anti-inflammatory diet. Add mixed green salad with toppings of almonds, tuna, slices of balsamic dressing and avocado in your lunch. It must be served with whole-grain crackers, minestrone soup with low sodium and a bowl of non-fat yogurt.

You can also have whole-wheat pita accompanied with grilled eggplant, hummus, onions and peppers and serve them with mixed berries, side salad and some walnuts.

You can include broccoli, carrots, garlic and ginger, bok choy with tofu or chicken and brown rice for a gluten-free anti-inflammatory lunch.

Snacks

In any diet plan, snacks are also very important. For this, include anti-inflammatory and healthy options like fresh veggies and fruits, nonfat Greek yogurt, unsalted nuts, whole-grain crackers with steamed edamame and nut butter. Snack calories must be less than 200 and you should avoid overeating.

Dinner

Add grilled salmon for dinner with roasted new potatoes and Brussels sprouts dipped on rosemary, olive oil and garlic. Spice them up with tofu curry or vegetable curry served with mixed green salad or on brown rice. Or you may stuff tortilla with chopped tomatoes, bean puree and lettuce and serve them with corn, salsa and spinach salad with walnuts.

CHAPTER 4

ANTI-INFLAMMATORY LIFESTYLE – THE BEST WAY TO SAY "NO" TO DISEASES

Arthritis, Heart Disease, Diabetes, Depression and Allergies – These diseases have one thing in common – **Inflammation**.

All of these diseases, and several others, are known as inflammatory diseases because they are caused due to whole body, chronic inflammation. There are several ads of latest drugs that claim to treat their symptoms. But, you can still choose to go with some scientifically-proven yet natural ways to control inflammation and prevent such diseases before they get worse. Before we jump on the benefits of anti-inflammatory lifestyle, here's why inflammation is taken so seriously.

Despite the strong and advanced healthcare system across the world, inflammation is getting worse. The diseases we have discussed above affected millions of people in the US alone.

- **Diabetes** – Around 24 million people in the US are suffering from this condition. By 2025, it is estimated to be around 50 million if it is not controlled.

- **Arthritis** – Around 20% of the US population, i.e. over 43 million are affected by this disease. By 2020, it is estimated to cross 60 million.

- **Obesity** – Over 2/3rd of adults are obese or overweight and around 1/3 of people are suffering from obesity.

- **Allergies** – It is another serious problem caused by inflammation.

- **Asthma** – Over 25 million people are suffering from asthma

- **Anxiety & Depression** – Over 18 million Americans are suffering from it

- **Alzheimer's disease** – Around 5 million people are affected in the US alone.

The Benefits of Anti-Inflammatory Lifestyle

The anti-inflammatory diet plan should be designed uniquely to fit with your genes to control inflammation in the entire body, lose weight and boost energy and set you free to live every moment of your life to the fullest. Foods, exercise and nutrition help us reduce inflammation in a natural way. It is one of the best and healthiest lifestyle approaches. Here are some of the best benefits of anti-inflammatory lifestyle -

Proactively Control Inflammation

People are often recommended to start anti-inflammatory diet plan who are suffering from the disease that is related to chronic inflammation. There are actually hundreds of autoimmune disorders and diseases which are related to inflammation, such as rheumatoid arthritis, Alzheimer's disease, osteoarthritis, cancer, Chrohn's Disease, eczema, diabetes, psoriasis, ulcers and stroke, to name a few. Inflammation has been concerned with age-related Alzheimer's disease, cognitive diseases, schizophrenia, and depression.

But with anti-inflammatory lifestyle, you can naturally reduce the risks of developing such diseases and control the conditions related to inflammation.

Enhanced Energy

The usual Western diet is loaded with sugary and refined foods which can spine our energy for a bit and we end up with less energy and sluggish lifestyle for long term. Unhealthy diet can also reduce our emotional energy which can prevent us thinking clearly and increase brain fog.

But anti-inflammatory diet includes the foods which are organically rich in fiber and polyphenols, such as vegetables, fruits, beans and nuts. We often get sustained energy by eating certain types of foods that are naturally fiber rich. Omega-3 rich fish and other lean protein sources are some of the best sources to provide enhanced energy. Fewer sugar crashes and spikes and lasting and sustained energy all day long are the great benefits of anti-inflammatory lifestyle.

Weight Loss

You can easily lose weight by following anti-inflammatory lifestyle. There are some people in a study who lost around 2 pounds of weight and around 0.5% of fat in a week. The best thing is that the anti-inflammatory diet plan is simple. It is not like traditional weight-loss plans. In fact, you can enjoy your favorite meals and feel satisfied and fuller after eating.

Kick Out Chronic Diseases

We have listed several chronic diseases above that are caused by inflammation. This way, anti-inflammatory lifestyle can help you prevent the associated risks. It can reduce metabolic syndrome by 44%.

Freedom to Enjoy Your Favorite Food

More often than not, we get bored with certain diets and we end up avoiding them. We often feel that we are losing something from our life every time when we have food. Such types of restrictive diets are not sustainable at all and we often end up feeling failed and quitting the existing diet.

But the best part of anti-inflammatory diet is that it is completely different from other annoying diet plans. We can easily add the foods we love in our diet. In addition, we feel fuller, satisfied and energized all the time. We can have more freedom to live every moment of our life more fully.

All the foods it includes are rich in fiber, protein, and vitamins. Only thing it restricts are fatty and unhealthy fast foods that we must strictly avoid. These foods increase inflammation in our body and make us vulnerable to several diseases. The anti-inflammatory lifestyle gives us freedom to choose the fruits and vegetables we love.

CHAPTER 5

CONTROLLING INFLAMMATION WITH HEALTHY DIET

Certain diets and foods are responsible to cause inflammation. But you can control the risk of inflammation and certain health problems like heart disease, Alzheimer's disease, psoriasis, diabetes, Crohn's disease and rheumatoid arthritis, by choosing the best anti-inflammatory foods and avoiding unhealthy foods that we will discuss later. So without wasting any time, let's starts with what anti-inflammatory foods you should start eating.

Anti-Inflammatory Foods To Eat

Switch to time-honored Mediterranean diet, such as whole grains, beans, fruits and vegetables and try to avoid a common American diet. The

Mediterranean diet contains foods that have high amount of Omega 3 acids and monounsaturated fat. Foods which are high in Trans Fats, sugar, refined starches and saturated fats are bad for your health. Instead, start having the following anti-inflammatory foods -

Colorful Fruits & Veggies

These foods are rich in antioxidants that help control inflammation, such as flavonoids and beta-carotene and Vitamins A, E and C. Choose bright colored vegetables and fruits because they have more antioxidants. Some of the nutritious options are apples, grapes, green leafy vegetables, berries, cherries, sweet potatoes and so on.

Whole Grains

There are refined grains contained in trade foods. But foods containing whole grains are rich in antioxidants and fiber. Oatmeal, whole wheat bread, whole-wheat pasta, and brown rice play a vital role in anti-inflammatory diet. Whole wheat pasta can help you reduce inflammation if you eat 2-3 servings every week.

Spices and Herbs

There are certain spices and herbs which can add taste and pleasure to your diet. In addition, they also improve your health because they have certain anti-inflammatory properties. Spices and herbs like cinnamon, cayenne peppers, basil, cloves, rosemary, ginger, mint, parsley, turmeric and oregano can reduce inflammation.

Polyunsaturated Fats

These are healthy fats which provide better protection to your heart health. These healthy fats are usually found in flax seeds, walnuts, corn oil, sunflower oil, flaxseed oil and soybean oil. There are certain fish like halibut, salmon, herring and sardines contain Omega-3 fat and polyunsaturated fats. They reduce inflammation and the risk of sudden heart attacks. Omega 3 acids help control the risk of arthritis and cancer.

Inflammation-Causing Foods to Avoid

In 2004, around 12.9 millions are died due to heart disease across the world, as stated by the World Health Organization. According to World Cancer Research Fund, the number of deaths occurred from cancer are estimated to around 8 million. The deadly combo of chronic inflammation – Cancer & Heart

Disease – is known to be the major cause that leads to such a great number of death cases in the world.

But you can still reduce the risk of cancer and heart disease with certain lifestyle changes by adopting foods that are healthy. You should cut down or avoid certain foods that lead to cause inflammation. Here is the list of foods you should beware of –

Sugars

Consuming excessive sugary items can cause tooth decay which also leads to inflammation, obesity, and serious diseases like Type 2 diabetes and metabolic syndrome. They are found in sweetened beverages like fruit drinks, soft drinks and some punches. Having a can of Diet Coke is equivalent to eating ten sugar cubes. Some sugary foods you should avoid are desserts, pastries, snacks and candies. When you see the labels, make sure that sugar is mentioned in several names like fructose, dextrose, corn syrup, maltose, golden syrup, and sucrose and sorghum syrup.

If you have a sweet tooth, try honey, stevia, or blackstrap molasses as flavorings instead. Certain foods with no added sugar and preservatives are healthy choices. You can go for dried or fresh fruits.

Basic Vegetable Cooking Oils

Some vegetable oils used for cooking at restaurants and homes are high in Omega 6 fatty acids. Foods have high omega-6 imbalanced fat can lead to inflammatory diseases like cancer and heart diseases. These fats are usually found in vegetable oils like cottonseed, grape seed, corn, safflower and sunflower. Replace these cooling oils and switch to extra virgin olive oil, macadamia oil, and various edible oils which have more balanced Omega-3 fatty acids.

Trans Fat

Trans fatty acids are known for increasing levels of unhealthy cholesterol and reducing levels of healthy cholesterol. They also lead to obesity, inflammation and resistance to insulin. They are widely found in fast foods, deep fried foods, and commercially baked foods and the items prepared with margarine, partly hydrogenated oil and vegetable shortening. Another major threat is commercially-made peanut butter. So, it is best to read the list of ingredients and check the labels to avoid foods that contain vegetable shortening and partly hydrogenated oil.

Dairy

Milk is a well-known allergen which can cause inflammatory responses like constipation, stomach distress, skin rashes, diarrhea, acne, breathing problems and hives in those who cannot digest it. Certain dairy and milk products contain deficiency of Omega 3 fatty acids. It is also important to avoid cookies, crackers, bread, cream sauces, cakes and boxed cereals which have hidden dairy content, along with cheese and butter. Instead, you can have unsweetened yogurt and kefir in moderation if you don't have allergy from milk.

Processed Meat and Red Meat

Red meat has a molecule "Neu5Gc" that we don't produce naturally. Our body develops antibodies to prevent Neu5Gc when we ingest it. And it leads to severe inflammatory response which is linked to heart disease and cancer. Basic red meats are lamb, beef and pork and processed meats are sausage, salami and ham.

CHAPTER 6

ADD THESE HERBS AND SPICES TO YOUR MEALS TO REDUCE INFLAMMATION

Certain herbs and spices have been used for years by all Ayurvedic and Chinese practitioners in order to cure all types of diseases because they have antioxidants and anti-inflammatory properties. Both oxidation and inflammation are closely linked to each other.

Nutrients are also capable to avoid inflammation in different ways. Just a ½ tsp of ground cinnamon has antioxidants equals to ½ cup of blueberries. Similarly, there are other spices and herbs that can help prevent inflammation –

Turmeric

Turmeric is the spice that has life-enhancing benefits. It has been used for centuries as Chinese and Ayurvedic medicine to cure almost every ailment like arthritis, liver disease, and immune disorders. According to some studies, turmeric has anti-inflammatory, antioxidant; antifungal, antibacterial, antiviral and anticancer properties and it can prevent several inflammatory diseases like diabetes, arthritis, allergies, and Alzheimer's disease.

The benefits of turmeric are endless and it has a potent antioxidant that drastically controls inflammation. It reduces the buildup of tumor cells and promotes insulin resistance. Turmeric also prevents the buildup of beta-amyloid plaques which lead to Alzheimer's disease. So, sprinkle some turmeric on your dishes and enjoy variety of health benefits.

Ginger

Like turmeric, ginger has also been used to cure pain and inflammation for centuries. It also soothes sore throats and muscles and prevents general fatigue and aches. It has shogauls, gingerols, and paradols to attack inflammation. 6-gingerol is a potent antioxidant found in ginger to prevent buildup of free radicals that cause pain and inflammation. Ginger can block several pain-causing chemicals related to arthritis. So, it is a best alternative to drugs.

In Asian dishes, it works really very well and you can add it on your tea to cure cold and sore throat. You can easily use ginger in certain foods and apply it to the painful joints directly for relief. You can easily use ginger in your foods or even apply it to the affected area directly.

Cloves

Cloves are rich in Eugenol and several anti-inflammatory properties. You can add it into your food and increase the taste. It can help control inflammation and trigger the effects of pro-inflammatory cytokines. Cloves are widely used in sweet baked goods. It can also be added on savory dishes like meats for added flavor. It can also be added on ginger tea. Cloves are very powerful spice and also have antifungal properties.

Sage

Sage has anti-inflammatory molecules like carnosol and carnosic acids that provide great health benefits and increase the aroma and flavor. It can also prevent neurological problems that are related to inflammation like Alzheimer's disease. The herb also increases focus and memory and reduces anxiety. Both carnosol and carnosic acid have anticancer and antioxidant properties. Sage can easily be used in sausages, winter squash and meat roasts. It also contains camphor which kills fungi and bacteria.

Cinnamon Sprinkles

Cinnamon has anti-inflammatory agents - cinnamyl aldehydes and cinnamic aldehyde. According to a 2013 study, adding cinnamon to the diet can help you reduce muscle pain. It is also helpful for people who have diabetes. But you need to ask your doctor before adding this herb to your food if you are diabetic patient. You can add it to your yogurt, hot cereal, tea or coffee to control inflammation.

Rosemary

It also contains carnosol and carnosic acids along with "rosemarinic acid" which is another anti-inflammatory compound. Both sage and rosemary improve the performance of superoxide dismutase which removes superoxide. It is a potent free radical which can cause chronic inflammation. Rosemary can be used to add taste in meats, roasted veggies and various cooked dishes.

CHAPTER 7

CHOOSING RIGHT COOKING OIL FOR YOUR ANTI-INFLAMMATORY DIET

Cooking oil is considered to be the most vital and basic need of cooking in every kitchen. But it is very important to choose the right cooking oil. You may visit any supermarket and find lots of bottles of cooking oils from various brands. There are wide ranges of cooking oils, i.e. from corn oils and refined soybean oils that are commonly used to premium and exotic oils like cold pressed coconut oils and extra virgin avocado oils.

Choosing the Best Cooking Oil

Here's what you should look for while picking the next cooking oil from the shelves –

Consider Omega 3 and Omega 6 Ratio

Both Omega 3 and Omega 6 fatty acids have PUFA (Polyunsaturated Fatty Acids) which is essential for your health. Some of these fats cannot be produced by our body. We have to add these fats on the food we eat daily. However, having excess of Omega 6 without having enough Omega 3 can lead to inflammation.

Omega 6 is more inflammatory than Omega 3 and foods that have higher level of Omega 6 than Omega 3 can produce pro-inflammatory compounds in your body.

Unfortunately, modern American diet is loaded with Omega 6 and lacks Omega 3 fatty acids because vegetable oils that contain high PUFA levels are used. Cooking oil must have Omega 6 Omega 3 ratio of 1:1 to 4:1. So, it is wise to look for cooking oils that have high Omega 3 and low Omega 6.

Choose Oils with Monounsaturated Fats

According to several studies, using cooking oils rich in monounsaturated fats like olive oil can help control risk of heart disease by increasing HDL levels (High Density Lipoprotein) and reducing LDL cholesterol levels (Low Density Lipoprotein).

Oleic acid is Omega 9 monounsaturated fatty acid which is known to be responsible to protect heart. It is found in olive oil. Olive oil also contains phytochemicals like oleuropein and hydroxytyrosol which play a vital role to protect our heart.

Beware of Cooking Oils Having High Polyunsaturated Fats

Oils that contain over 50% of polyunsaturated fatty acids are likely to be unstable. The oxidation process of PUFA starts when oil is exposed to light, air and heat and is extracted. It breaks down purity of oil and forms free radicals. When oil is heated, degeneration gets worse. Higher temperature forms more inflammatory oxidation. So, never heat extra virgin, unrefined PUFA. However, some oils like flaxseed oils are great source of Omega 3 fatty acids.

Consider the Process of Extraction

Certain commercially refined vegetable oils, such as corn oils and soybean oils are basically extracted with harmful solvents like hexane. When short ingestion of less chemical don't cause any issue, but long term ingestion may affect. So, consider the presence of cooking oil in all foods you eat daily. Consider choosing food grade oils that have been mechanically extracted. These types of oils are basically labeled as 'expeller-pressed' or 'cold-pressed'.

Telltale Signs To Determine The Freshness Of Your Cooking Oil

After deciding the best type of oil to use, next important thing is checking out the freshness. Only nutrition and quality are not important to buy cooking oil. It doesn't matter how healthy any oil be. Once it's gone worse, you could put your life at risk. Here's how to determine the freshness of oil -

Production Date – Pick a bottle of oil which is closer to production or harvest date. The more the oil gets old on the shelves, the more nutrition it loses. Also buy the amount of oil that can completely be used within half a year.

Nitrogen Seal – Oxygen is a major culprit that makes oil lose its freshness. Some makers replace air on the container with oxygen. Unlike oxygen, nitrogen keeps oil fresher for longer. But once the seal is broken and container is opened, oil remains no longer secured and starts losing its freshness. So, it is better to use up the oil as faster as you can.

Color of Container – When oil is exposed to light, it loses up freshness faster. So it is wise to avoid the oil which is stored in transparent, clear container or bottle. Instead, go for the one which is stored in green/dark amber glass bottle or tin.

Storage Temperature – If the temperature is higher, the oil will go rancid. Since most of the oils are kept in cool air condition, it is not a problem at all. But at home, it might be an issue because it is usually stored near the stove. The stove releases high heat that shortens the life of oil and destroys its goodness. So, it is better to store the oil in dark, cool place.

Recommended Anti-Inflammatory Cooking Oils

Extra Virgin Olive Oil

When it comes to MUFA or Monounsaturated Fatty Acids, most of us think of olive oil. Over 70% of fats are MUFA in olive oil and it is the de facto choice for most of us. Olive oil comes in different varieties. But cold-pressed, organic, extra virgin olive oil is the best variety.

It will not just have phyto-chemicals with antioxidants, it will also have richer and stronger flavor. It has high amount of Omega 9 MUFA and unique taste. But the problem is that it is not suitable for cooking in high temperature. It is used on cold dishes and added just after turning off the gas.

Pure Ghee

It is a typical clarified butter which is widely used in India and various countries of South Asia. It has great ratio of Omega 6 to Omega 3. It has high amount of saturated fat and it doesn't oxidize with ease. It has very low lactose and it is good choice for those who have allergy to lactose.

It has low levels of polyunsaturated fats and has rich buttery aroma and taste. It doesn't oxidize with ease and has high smoke point. So, you can easily use it to cook at high temperature.

Avocado Oil

It is usually pressed from avocado's pulp instead of its seed. It has high smoke point, i.e. up to 204 Deg. C (400 Deg F), if it is in extra virgin form. Refined avocado oil has smoke point of up to 271 Deg. C (520 Deg F). It is rich in Omega 9 monounsaturated fat and has high polyhydroxylated and phytosterols fatty alcohols which are quite anti-inflammatory. It is good for high temperature cooking like high heat baking and Stir Frying.

CHAPTER 8

ANTI-INFLAMMATORY INGREDIENTS YOU MUST HAVE IN YOUR KITCHEN

Year after year, more and more people are using natural ingredients to cure common health problems. Several common ingredients in your kitchen provide great health benefits you may not know. These ingredients provide something beyond their basic purpose of making your food delicious. They are providing a lot of health benefits, ranging from minor to major. Here are some of the basic kitchen ingredients that act as medicines –

Ginger

Ginger has antispasmodic, anti-inflammatory, antiseptic, antifungal, antiviral and antibacterial properties. It is an effective and natural painkiller. Ginger is really a great source of magnesium, potassium, phosphorous, vitamins A, B-Complex, C and E, and zinc. Ginger can be used to cure indigestion, upset stomach, nausea, heartburn and motion sickness, arthritis pain and common body pain, cough, cold and various respiratory problems, menstrual cramps and fever.

Turmeric

For cooking, turmeric is a widely-used spice for taste. It also has antibacterial, antiseptic, antioxidant and anti-inflammatory properties. Turmeric can be used to disinfect common burns and cuts and cough, common cold, arthritis, joint pain, acne, bruised skin, pimples and several stomach problems. It can also reduce the risk of liver damage due to alcohol or drug abuse and also prevents Alzheimer's disease. It has antioxidant properties to treat different kinds of cancer, like colon cancer, breast cancer, leukemia and lung cancer.

Cinnamon

Cinnamon has carminative, anti-inflammatory, antiseptic, antioxidant, and anti-flatulent properties. It is also rich in minerals like calcium, potassium, iron, manganese, zinc, copper, niacin, Vitamin A and pyridoxine. Cinnamon is widely used to cure flatulence, common cold, heartburn, indigestion, diarrhea, nausea, menstrual cramps and arthritis pain.

By having cinnamon regularly, you can easily control Type-2 diabetes and blood sugar level. It also helps reduce cholesterol level and minimize the risk of heart disease of several types. However, it must not be consumed in excess as it may lead to toxicity.

Garlic

It is also known as superfood because of its diaphoretic, stimulant, anti-bacterial, diuretic, expectorant, antiviral, antifungal and antiseptic properties. Garlic is loaded with nutrients and vitamins like potassium, protein, zinc, calcium etc. Garlic can cure chronic bronchitis, cough, hoarseness, sore throat, asthma, sinus problems, indigestion, ear infection, colic, stomach ache, toothache, ringworm and bug bites. It can be helpful to prevent strokes and lower cholesterol levels.

Honey

It has antifungal, antiviral, anti-parasitic, and antiseptic properties. It is also rich in several essential minerals and vitamins like potassium, calcium, copper, sodium, iron, sulfur, manganese, phosphate and zinc. Honey can help cure throat irritation, cough, canker sores, laryngitis, and morning sickness, eczema, and stomach ulcers. It also relieves minor wounds, burns and infections. It is also loaded with carbohydrates to boost athletic performance, reduce muscle fatigue and improve endurance.

Lemon

Lemon has a lot of antioxidant properties which can help boost immunity. It has several nutrients like folate and vitamin C. Lemon ha a lot of medicinal uses to cure throat infections, headaches, indigestion, dental problems, constipation, bug bites, dandruff, rheumatism, arthritis, and internal bleeding. It is helpful to reduce high blood pressure, lose weight, and prevent kidney stones. With regular use, lemon can be helpful to avoid several problems like heart disease, strokes and cancer of several types.

Onion

It has great antiseptic, anti-inflammatory, antimicrobial, antibiotic and carminative benefits. It is also rich in Vitamins B1, B6, C and K, calcium, chromium, biotin, dietary fiber and folic acid. Onion is also very effective to cure cough, common cold, pneumonia, chronic bronchitis, asthma and hay fever. It also effectively combats nausea, stomach upset and diarrhea. It also plays vital role in controlling risk of different types of cancer.

Anti Inflammatory Meals To Eat

Inflammation and chronic diseases are closely related to each other because of inactive lifestyle and poor diet. Inflammation causes cancer, heart diseases, strokes, arthritis etc. as we have discussed so many times earlier.

No matter you are eating no carb, low-carb, vegan, vegetarian, Neanderthal or Mediterranean, here are some of the delicious recipes for breakfast, lunch, dinner, dessert and snacks that can support your anti-inflammatory lifestyle –

Recipe for Breakfast

Citrus Frittata

Yields – 4 to 6 servings

Ingredients

- 12 Organic Eggs
- ½ Coconut milk
- 2 tbsp extra virgin olive oil or coconut oil
- ½ tsp sea salt or according to taste
- 1 cup arugula or spinach
- Sautéed mushrooms or any other vegetable – ½ cup
- Finely chopped red onion – 1

How to Prepare?

- Preheat your oven up to 375 Deg. F
- Whisk coconut milk and eggs with salt and keep aside.
- Heat up the pan on medium-high level with coconut oil and fry the onions until they get transparent. Add any vegetable or mushroom and stir fry until they turn soft. Add spinach and fold on the mixture of veggies until they get wilted. After removing veggies from pan, set them aside.
- Turn the heat level down and add more coconut oil when needed. Add eggs and shake the pan to spread the mixture properly. Cook in medium-low heat for at least 5 minutes and spread the eggs with spatula from the corners to the center. Arrange the veggie mixture on the top.
- Stir it on the oven and cook for five minutes more until it turns slightly browned. Remove it from the oven. Slide the frittata on the large plate and place the plate on the pan and hold

both of them together so the partly cooked frittata can be dropped on the plate. Slide it back on the pan and place it back on the oven to cook for 3 to 4 minutes more. You can serve it with vinaigrette or salad.

Recipe for Lunch

Steamy Hot Quinoa Salad & Cashews
Yields – 4 Servings

Ingredients
- Dried Quinoa – 1 Cup (Properly rinsed)
- Red Onion (Finely Chopped) – ½
- Carrot/Apple (Thinly Chopped) – 1 Cup
- 1 Lime for Juicing
- Extra-Virgin Olive Oil – 1 tbsp
- Agave or Honey – 2 tbsp
- Mango (Chopped) – 1 Large
- Sea Salt – for taste

- Mint (Finely Chopped) – ¼ cup
- Avocado (Finely Sliced or Chopped) – 1
- Ginger (Finely Chopped) – ½ inch piece
- Black pepper (Freshly Grounded) – for taste
- Cashews (roughly chopped) – 1 Cup
- Romaine Lettuce or any green vegetable you like (Coarsely Chopped) – 3 Cups

How to Prepare?

1. Boil 2 cups of water in saucepan at medium heat. Add quinoa and cover it for 15 to 20 minutes in low heat. Put it aside and let it cool.

2. Sprinkle the apple/carrot and chopped red onion in large bowl. Mix them with honey, lime juice and olive oil. Add the mango and cooled, cooked quinoa to bowl and mix well. Stir in cilantro,

mint, salt, ginger and pepper for taste. Add cashews and sliced avocado for garnishing. Add the mixture on the greens and serve at moderate temperature or chilled.

Recipe for Dinner

Black Sesame Salmon with Consommé & Bok Choy

Yields – 2 to 3 servings

Ingredients
- Wild Salmon (pound pieces) – 2 Quarter
- Thinly sliced lime – 1
- Seafood stock – 3 cups
- Whole black peppercorns – 10
- Lime juice
- Bok Choy – 2 heads
- Pepper and salt – for taste
- Black sesame seeds (toasted) for garnishing

Note - This recipe can also be prepared with chicken. All you need to poach a few skinless, boneless, organic breasts for around 15 minutes, and keep it aside in broth covered for 15 minutes extra to steam.

How to Prepare?

- Stir in limes, peppercorns, and seafood stock to the heavy pot or deep skillet on high heat and boil them and reduce the heat immediately. Cook the mixture for 5 minutes approx.

- Season salmon with pepper and salt and lower the heat gently to simmer and cover the filets for at least ¾ parts. Bring down the heat gently to simmer and cover and cook it for around 5 to 6 minutes until salmon is thick properly. Remove salmon and keep aside on the plate lined by towel.

- Turn Up the heat to medium and then simmer. Add the Bok Choy and cook it for around 3 minutes until they turn soft. Remove them from the liquid.

- Turn up the heat to medium and keep cooking the broth for 3 minutes more. Turn off the heat and add lime juice on it and turn the heat off.

- Split the salmon and Bok Choy between two plain bowls. And add around ½ or ¼ cup of broth on each bowl. Add black sesame seeds over it.

Recipe for Dessert

Choco Shake with Cherry
Yields – 1 to 2 Glass

Ingredients
- Frozen dark cherries – ½ cup

- Unprocessed, unsweetened cocoa powder – 1 tbsp
- Almond, coconut or flax milk – 1 cup
- Pure vanilla extract – ½ tsp
- Ice cubes

How to Prepare?

All you need to put all of these ingredients in blender and process them until they turn smooth.

Recipe for Snacking

Carrot Muffins
Yields – 12 pieces

Ingredients
- Rice Milk – 1 Cup
- Egg – 1
- Canola Oil – 4 tablespoon
- Quinoa flour – 2 Cups
- Guar Gum – 1 Teaspoon

- Flaxseed Meal – 1 Tablespoon
- Baking Powder – 3 teaspoon
- Cinnamon – 1 teaspoon
- Salt – for taste
- Brown sugar – ¼ cup
- Organic carrots – 1 cup
- Raisins – ¼ cup

Instructions

- Preheat the oven to at least 400 Degree Fahrenheit (200 Deg. C)
- Mix the rice milk, egg, and canola oil and add dry ingredients in another bowl.
- Mix both dry and liquid ingredients until they get blended. Don't overly mix them. Fold in raisins and grated carrots.
- Fill in 12 muffin cups with around 2/3rd full of batter and bake it for 20 minutes.

DISCLAIMER

The book "Anti-Inflammatory Diet" contains information that can be helpful to cure and diagnose any health issue. Not all exercise and diet plans can be suitable for everyone. So, before starting any diet, starting any weight-loss or fitness program, or taking medication of any kind, you must ask your doctor or medical professional. Neither the publisher nor the author shall be responsible for any kind of problem related to this book.

This publication includes the ideas and opinions from the author. The book is designed to provide some insightful and detailed information about the particular subject matter. If you need personal advice or help, you should consult a professional. The publisher and the author disclaim any liability or responsibility, for risk or loss of any kind, associated with the accuracy of content in this book.

All Rights Reserved

ABOUT AUTHOR

I am Cheryl Barnhart, a housewife, a mother, a writer, and a dietitian. I love cooking and eating a lot. I keep on reading various cookbooks, recipe guides, and food books. After reading them, I become so expert in cooking, that I started to write my own books. My husband and family encouraged me a lot in writing, and started with my first book, which was on "Beer Brewing At Home". It got a good response, so then after I wrote another book on "Eat Nourish And Grow". Now I am working more on cooking and dieting books. To get updates about all my newly release books follow me and share your views with me....